A French book written and translated in 2023
by Fabien Bear.

HEALTH

# Intermittent fasting

A effective way to lose weight
& live longer

**FABIEN BEAR**

# table of contents


**INTRODUCTION** 7

**I. Understanding Intermittent Fasting** 11
What is Intermittent Fasting ?
Different Types of Intermittent Fasting
How does it work ?

**II. The Benefits** 15
Weight and Fat Loss
Improved Metabolic Health
Reduced Risk of Chronic Diseases
Better Cognition and Concentration
Improved Longevity

**III. How to Practice Intermittent Fasting ?** 21
Different Intermittent Fasting Methods
How to Start Intermittent Fasting
How to Plan Your Meals During Fasting and Non-Fasting Periods
How to Eat Healthily During Non-Fasting Periods

**IV. Possible Side Effects** 27
Common Side Effects and How to Avoid Them
Contraindications of Intermittent Fasting

**VI. Myths and Realities**                                    31

Misconceptions about Intermittent Fasting

Realities of this Practice


**CONCLUSION**                                                35

# Introduction

# How has intermittent fasting become popular?

Intermittent fasting is a practice that involves alternating periods of fasting and normal eating. This practice has become increasingly popular in recent years, with many advocates claiming that it can help with weight loss, improve metabolic health, increase energy, and reduce the risk of chronic diseases.

In this first part of our book, we will explore the history of intermittent fasting and the reasons why it has become so popular today. We will also examine the potential health benefits that have been associated with this practice.

# The History of Intermittent Fasting

Intermittent fasting is not a new practice, and it has been practiced in different cultures for centuries. For example, religious practices such as Ramadan in Islam, Lent in Christianity, and Yom Kippur in Judaism are examples of intermittent fasting.

However, it is only recently that this practice has become popular in the context of health and wellness. The first research on the effects of intermittent fasting on health was conducted in the 1940s and 1950s, but the practice remained relatively unknown for decades.

# Potential Health Benefits

In recent years, more and more research has been conducted to study the effects of intermittent fasting on health. The results have shown that this practice can have many health benefits, including weight and body fat loss, improved metabolic health, reduced risk of chronic diseases such as diabetes, cardiovascular disease, and cancer, as well as improved cognition and longevity.

In the rest of this book, we will explore in detail the different ways of practicing intermittent fasting, the pros and cons, contraindications, common myths, and strategies for incorporating this practice into your daily life.

By learning to fast responsibly and understanding the many health benefits, you may be able to discover the potential of intermittent fasting for your own life and overall well-being.

# Understanding Intermittent Fasting

In this first part, we will explore the basics of intermittent fasting. We will see what it is, how it works, and the different types of intermittent fasting.

## What is intermittent fasting ?

Intermittent fasting is a practice that involves alternating between periods of fasting and periods of normal eating. There are many ways to practice intermittent fasting, and fasting periods can vary in duration and frequency.
Most people practice intermittent fasting by limiting their daily feeding window to about 8 hours a day, practicing a 16-hour fast. This means they eat during an 8-hour window and fast for 16 hours.

## The different types of intermittent fasting.

There are several ways to practice intermittent fasting, each with different rules.
Here are some of the most popular types of intermittent fasting:
Daily intermittent fasting: also known as "16/8 fasting," this type of fasting involves fasting for 16 hours and eating within an 8-hour window each day.

- The 5:2 fasting: This method involves eating normally for 5 days a week and limiting calories to around 500-600 per day for the remaining 2 days.

- 24-hour fasting: This method involves fasting for 24 hours, one to two times per week.

- Alternate-day fasting: This method involves fasting every other day. During fasting days, only low-calorie liquids are allowed.

# How it works ?

LIntermittent fasting can help with weight loss by creating a calorie deficit and increasing insulin sensitivity, which can reduce the risk of type 2 diabetes. During fasting, the body transitions from a state of digestion to a state of fasting, allowing the body to burn stored fats for energy. This can help reduce body fat and improve body composition.

In summary, intermittent fasting can have beneficial effects on health, including reducing the risk of chronic diseases such as cardiovascular disease, cancer, and Alzheimer's disease. Research has also shown that intermittent fasting can improve cognition, brain function, and lifespan.

# Benefits

In this section, we will explore the benefits of intermittent fasting, such as weight loss, improvement in metabolic health, reduction in the risk of chronic diseases, improvement in cognition and concentration, and improvement in longevity.

# Weight and fat loss

Intermittent fasting is an effective method for losing weight and body fat. By creating a calorie deficit, intermittent fasting can help burn stored fat for energy. It can aid in fat loss by forcing the body to use fat reserves to produce energy. It can also improve the body's ability to use insulin by increasing sensitivity to this hormone. Insulin is responsible for regulating blood sugar by allowing cells to take in glucose from the blood and use it to produce energy. When insulin sensitivity is reduced, cells do not respond properly to this hormone and glucose remains in the blood, which can lead to health problems such as type 2 diabetes.
By increasing insulin sensitivity, intermittent fasting can help reduce insulin resistance and improve blood sugar regulation.
Intermittent fasting can lead to an increase in the production of certain hormones such as growth hormone and adrenaline, which are involved in regulating fat and carbohydrate metabolism.
It can also stimulate the production of norepinephrine, a hormone that can help burn fat.

## Improvement of metabolic health.

Intermittent fasting can improve metabolic health by reducing blood sugar, blood pressure, and blood lipid levels such as cholesterol and triglycerides. Blood pressure can be regulated by reducing the amount of salt and fluids in the body, as well as increasing the production of nitric oxide, which helps to relax blood vessels. By reducing these metabolic risk factors, intermittent fasting can help prevent chronic diseases such as cardiovascular disease and diabetes.

## Reduced risk of chronic diseases

Intermittent fasting can:
- Reduce the risk of chronic diseases, including cardiovascular diseases, cancer, and Alzheimer's disease. It can help to reduce inflammation and oxidative stress, which are common risk factors for these chronic diseases.

- Assist in reducing inflammation, which is associated with the development of many chronic diseases, by regulating levels of certain hormones and increasing the production of anti-inflammatory molecules

- Stimulate the production of growth hormones, which are important for cellular repair and regeneration.

# Improved cognition and concentration

Intermittent fasting can improve cognition and concentration by increasing the production of neurotrophic factors, which are proteins that promote the growth and survival of neurons. In addition, intermittent fasting can stimulate the production of BDNF, a neurotrophic factor that is important for brain function and memory.

BDNF stands for brain-derived neurotrophic factor, and it plays a crucial role in the development, growth, and maintenance of neurons in the brain. Studies have shown that BDNF levels increase during periods of fasting, which can lead to improved cognitive function, including better memory and learning ability. In addition to BDNF, intermittent fasting can also increase the production of other neurotrophic factors, such as FGF-2 and VEGF, which have been shown to promote the growth of new brain cells and blood vessels in the brain.

# Improvement of longevity

Intermittent fasting has been shown to increase longevity by upregulating the production of sirtuins, a family of proteins that play important roles in regulating metabolism and promoting longevity. Sirtuins are involved in a number of cellular processes, including DNA repair, energy metabolism, and inflammation. By promoting the production of sirtuins, intermittent fasting can help to reduce oxidative and inflammatory damage, which are both major contributors to aging and age-related diseases.

Additionally, studies have shown that intermittent fasting can improve the functioning of mitochondria, the energy-producing organelles within cells, which can also contribute to improved longevity.

# How to Practice Intermittent Fasting ?

In this section, we will show you how to practice intermittent fasting safely and effectively. We will explore the different methods of intermittent fasting, how to start intermittent fasting, how to plan your meals during fasting and non-fasting periods, and how to eat well during non-fasting periods.

## The different methods of intermittent fasting

Different methods of intermittent fasting involve different periods of fasting and non-fasting.

The most common methods are:

- 16/8 fasting: 16 hours of fasting and an 8-hour eating period. It is considered one of the easiest to follow and can help with weight loss, improve insulin sensitivity, and reduce inflammation.

- 24-hour fasting: 24 hours of fasting. It can help reduce inflammation and improve heart health by lowering triglyceride and LDL (bad cholesterol) levels.

- Alternate day fasting: one day of fasting followed by one day of non-fasting. It can help with weight loss and improve metabolic health by reducing blood sugar, blood pressure, and blood lipid levels.

- The 5:2 fasting: five days of non-fasting followed by two days of fasting. It can help with weight loss, improve heart health, and reduce inflammation.

## How to start intermittent fasting

It's important to start intermittent fasting gradually, slowly increasing the duration and frequency of your fasting periods.
It's also important to consult with your doctor before starting intermittent fasting if you have any health issues or if you're taking medication.

## How to plan your meals during fasting and non-fasting periods.

It is important to plan your meals during the non-fasting periods to ensure that you eat healthy and nutritious foods that support your body during intermittent fasting. During the fasting periods, it is important to drink plenty of water to avoid dehydration.

## How to eat well during non-fasting periods

It is important to eat healthy and nutritious foods during the non-fasting periods to support your body and maximize the benefits of intermittent fasting. Healthy foods to include in your diet include vegetables, fruits, lean proteins, whole grains, and healthy fats.

Examples of healthy and nutritious foods to include in your diet during the non-fasting periods are:

- Vegetables: spinach, broccoli, carrots, peppers, cauliflower, kale, salad, tomatoes, etc.

- Fruits: berries, apples, oranges, bananas, grapefruits, mangoes, etc.

Lean proteins: chicken, turkey, fish, tofu, beans, lentils, etc.

- Whole grains: brown rice, quinoa, oats, whole grain bread, whole grain pasta, etc.

- Healthy fats: nuts, seeds, olive oil, avocado, salmon, etc.

# Possible side effects

BAlthough intermittent fasting is generally considered safe for most people, there may be potential side effects.

In this section, we will examine the common side effects of intermittent fasting and how to avoid them. We will also address the contraindications of intermittent fasting.

## Common side effects and how to avoid them.

Intermittent fasting can lead to hunger and fatigue as the body adjusts to a new eating pattern. This is because the body is used to receiving food at certain times, and when it doesn't receive it, it can cause feelings of hunger and fatigue. Headaches and dizziness may also occur due to changes in blood sugar levels.

Constipation can be a result of dehydration, which can happen when someone is fasting and not drinking enough water. To avoid this, it is important to drink plenty of water and other fluids during fasting periods.

Irritability may occur due to changes in hormone levels and hunger, but it is typically temporary and can be managed through self-care practices like meditation or relaxation techniques.

It is important to note that these side effects are generally mild and short-lived, and many people do not experience any side effects at all. However, if someone experiences severe or persistent side effects, they should consult with a healthcare professional.

# *The contraindications of intermittent fasting*

Intermittent fasting may not be appropriate for everyone.

Certain groups of people should avoid intermittent fasting:
- Pregnant or breastfeeding women
- Children
- People with a history of eating disorders
- People with type 1 or type 2 diabetes who require insulin treatment
- People with liver or kidney disorders
- People with thyroid disorders

For pregnant or breastfeeding women, fasting can lead to nutritional deficiencies that can harm the health of the mother and the baby.

Children have high energy requirements and need regular meals to support their growth and development.

People with eating disorders may have a distorted relationship with food and fasting may trigger unhealthy behaviors. Intermittent fasting can also affect blood sugar levels and medication dosages in people with diabetes, liver, or kidney disorders.

In addition, people with thyroid disorders may be more sensitive to changes in metabolism and should consult with their healthcare provider before attempting intermittent fasting.

The myths & realities

Intermittent fasting has gained popularity in recent years, but there are also many myths and misconceptions circulating about it.

In this section, we will examine the myths and realities of intermittent fasting.

# The misconceptions about intermittent fasting

There are several misconceptions about intermittent fasting, including:

- Intermittent fasting leads to muscle loss: In reality, intermittent fasting may even help preserve muscle mass, especially if you exercise regularly.

- Intermittent fasting is dangerous: Intermittent fasting can be safe for most people if done responsibly and with the advice of your doctor.

- Intermittent fasting slows down metabolism: In reality, intermittent fasting can help improve metabolism by reducing inflammation and increasing insulin sensitivity.

# The realities of this practice

The realities of intermittent fasting are as follows:
- Intermittent fasting can help with weight loss: Intermittent fasting can help create a calorie deficit, which is necessary for weight loss.

- Intermittent fasting can help improve metabolic health: Intermittent fasting can help reduce blood sugar levels, improve insulin sensitivity, and reduce inflammation.

- Intermittent fasting is not suitable for everyone: Intermittent fasting may not be suitable for pregnant or breastfeeding women, children, individuals with eating disorders, individuals with type 1 or type 2 diabetes requiring insulin, individuals with liver or kidney disorders, and individuals with thyroid disorders.

# Conclusion

# *Integrating intermittent fasting into your lifestyle*

Intermittent fasting can offer numerous health benefits, including weight loss, improved metabolic health, decreased risk of chronic diseases, better cognition and concentration, and improved longevity. However, it is important to understand the different methods of intermittent fasting, how to practice it safely, and how to avoid common side effects.

If you are considering trying intermittent fasting, it is important to consult with your doctor to ensure it is suitable for your health status and to plan a program that fits your lifestyle. It is also important to educate yourself on what foods to consume during non-fasting periods to avoid compensating for missed calories during fasting periods.

Finally, research on intermittent fasting is still ongoing, and new developments may bring new discoveries about its health benefits. As such, it is important to stay informed about the latest research and to continue exploring the benefits of intermittent fasting for overall health improvement."

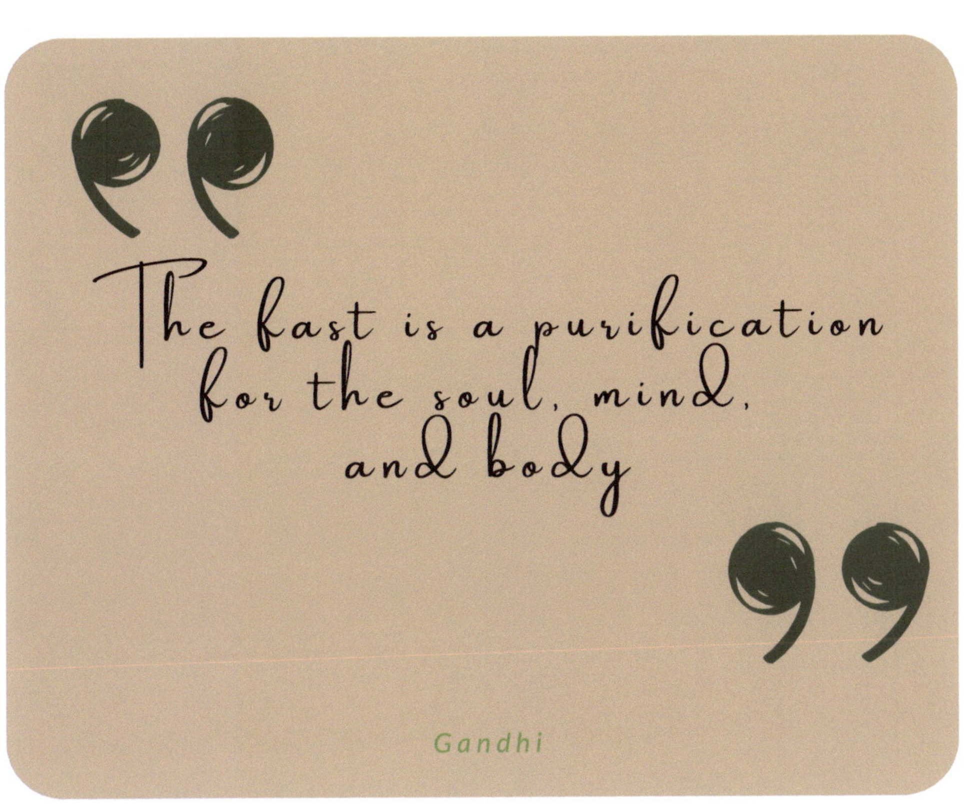



Gandhi

# Thanks !



@@fabien_bear_coaching

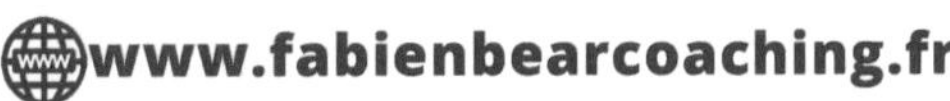
www.fabienbearcoaching.fr

www.ingramcontent.com/pod-product-compliance
Lightning Source LLC
Chambersburg PA
CBHW041808260726
48664CB00036B/1491